CRYSTAL HEALING

Revealed! The Exciting Secret to Using Powerful Crystals to Awaken Your Chakras, Boost Your Energy and Transform Your Life

Charice Kiernan

© **Copyright 2020 by Charice Kiernan – All rights reserved.**

In no way is it legal to reproduce, duplicate, or transmit any part of this document in either electronic means or in printed format. Recording of this publication is strictly prohibited and any storage of this document is not allowed unless with written permission from the publisher.

The information provided herein is stated to be truthful and consistent, in that any liability, in terms of inattention or otherwise, by any usage or abuse of any policies, processes, or directions contained within is the solitary and utter responsibility of the recipient reader. Under no circumstances will any legal responsibility or blame be held against the author for any reparation, damages, or monetary loss due to the information herein, either directly or indirectly.

The information herein is offered for informational purposes solely, and is universal as so. The presentation of the information is without contract or any type of guarantee assurance.

Medical Disclaimer: The ideas and suggestions contained in this book are not intended as a substitute for consulting with your physician. All matters regarding your health require medical supervision.

Legal Disclaimer: all photos used in this book are either in the public domain or licensed for commercial use.

ERRORS

Please contact me if you find any errors.

I have taken every effort to ensure the quality and correctness of this book. However, after going over the book draft time and again, I sometimes don't see the forest for the trees anymore :).

If you notice any errors, I would really appreciate it if you could contact me directly before taking any other action. This allows me to quickly fix it.

Errors: errors@charicekiernan.com

REVIEWS

Reviews and feedback help improve this book and myself as an author.

If you enjoy this book, I would greatly appreciate it if you were able to take a few moments to share your opinion and post a review online.

ENQUIRIES & FEEDBACK

For any general feedback about the book, please feel free to contact me at this email address: info@charicekiernan.com

By The Same Author

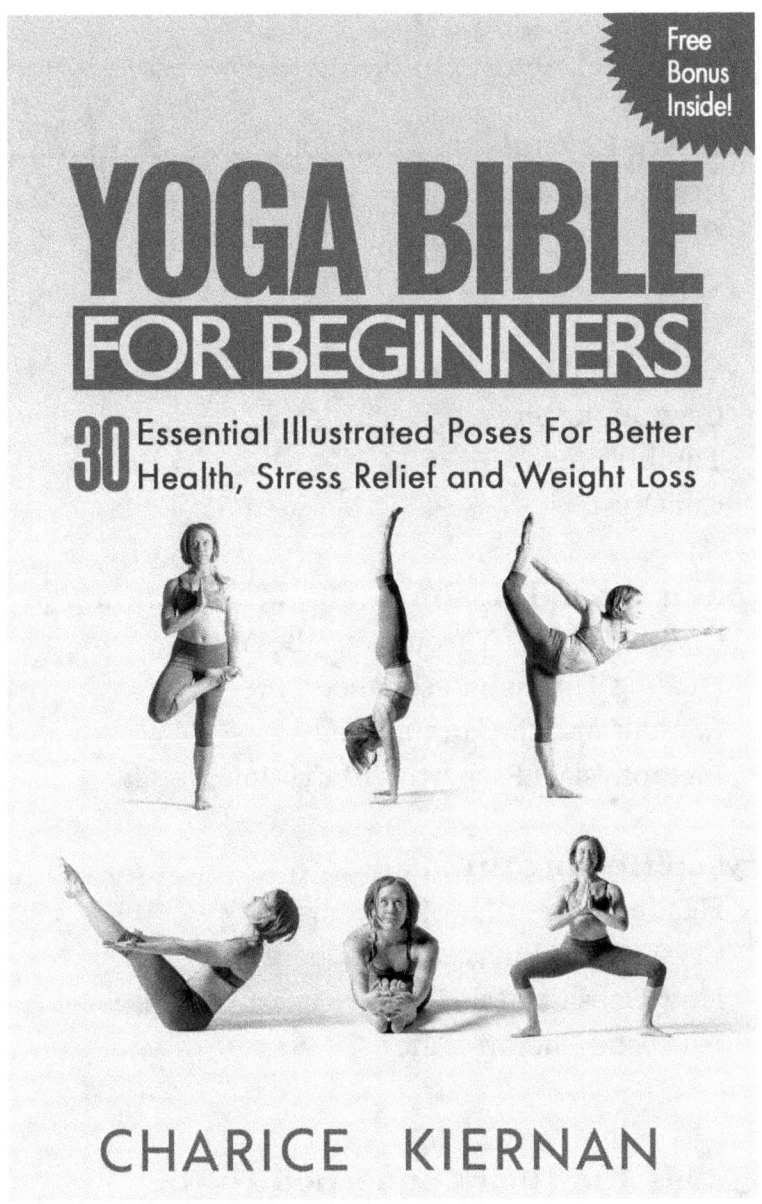

Table of Contents

Introduction..10

1. What Are Crystals?...14
    Crystallization
    Crystals are Different from Rocks and Glass
    Crystals Come in Many Different Shapes
    Crystal Families
    Crystal Habits
    Crystal Clusters
    Tumble Stones
    Cut Crystals

2. What is Crystal Healing....................................22
    Crystal Healing Throughout the Ages
    Healing Through Resonance
    Crystals and the Human Body
    Metaphysical Properties of Crystals

3. Crystal Healing 101...28
    Healing Properties of Crystals
    Crystals Are Energetically Charged
    How Does Crystal Healing Therapy Work
    Is Crystal Therapy Safe?

4. Crystals And Their Connection To The Chakras..36

Laws of Correspondence and Resonance
How These Laws Connect to the Chakras
Crystals and Their Effect on Chakras
The Root Chakra – Muladhara
The Sacral Chakra – Svadisthana
The Navel Chakra - Manipura
The Heart Chakra – Anahata
The Throat Chakra – Vishuddha
The Third Eye Chakra - Ajna
The Crown Chakra - Sahasrara

5. Eight Essential Healing Crystals..........................48
Clear Quartz
Rose Quartz
Citrine
Amethyst
Hematite
Fluorite
Black Tourmaline
Amazonite

6. Buying Crystals: Online or in a Store?................54
Buying a Crystal in a Store
Buying a Crystal Online

7. Five Tips to Ensure You Get the Most Out of Your Crystals..58
Tip 1: Do Your Research
Tip 2: Feel the Emerging Energy from the Crystal
Tip 3: Program your Crystals
Tip 4: Cleanse the Crystals

Tip 5: Experiment With Different Ways of Using the Crystals

8. How to Use These Crystals.....................62
Wearing Crystals on Your Body
Keeping Crystals Under Your Pillow
Using Crystals When Taking a Bath
Meditating with Crystals
Making Crystal Essences

9. Crystal Healing For Specific Conditions.............68
Headaches
Sleeplessness/Insomnia
Lack of Energy
Lack of Libido
Blood Circulation Disorders
Difficulty with Studying and Concentration
Healing the Mind
Crystal Healing and Love

10: Cleansing Your Crystals........................78
Smudging
Moonlight Clearing
Burying
Sacred Breath
Cool Water
Programming Your Crystals After the Cleanse

Final Words...86

BONUS CHAPTER: What is Yoga............................88
    The History of Yoga
    Modern Yoga

Did You Like This Book?...96

About The Author..,,98

Introduction

Thank you for picking up this book: *'Crystal Healing: Revealed! The exciting secret to using powerful crystals to awaken your chakras, boost your energy and transform your life.'*

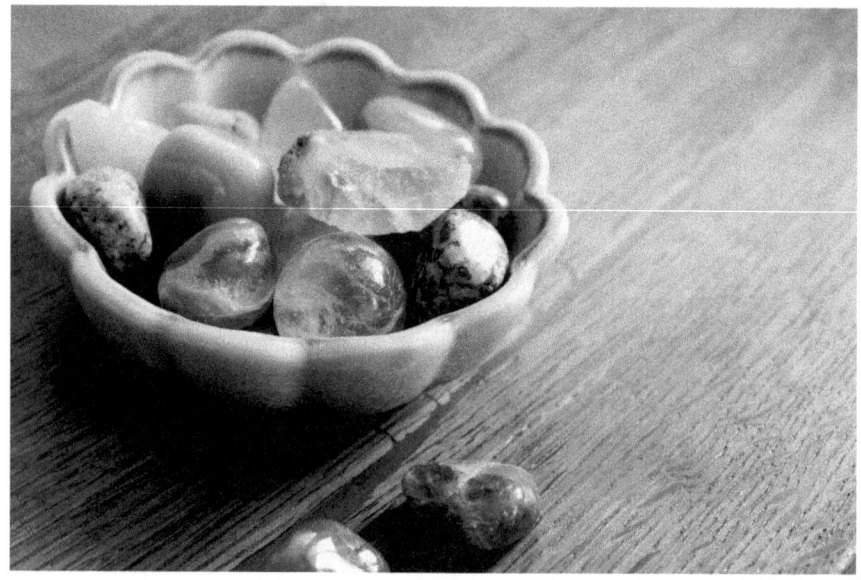

Welcome the wondrous world of crystals and their healing properties!

Crystals come in many different shapes and sizes, but they all share one fascinating quality: each crystal is charged with a unique and stable energy vibration. They can transform, amplify and transmit energy perfectly. For this reason, crystals are used in so many electrical devices used today.

What do a video console, electric guitar, phone and laptop have in common? You guessed it: they all, in one way or the other, rely on the crystals they have inside to function!

However, with all these technological applications, we may lose sight of crystals' most promising use: to heal ourselves.

Ancient civilizations across time have known about the secret power embedded in crystals. From the Egyptians, to the Mayans, Indian tribes and the Chinese medicine tradition: although they did not have access to the internet to contact each other, or find the information you now have in front of you, still they all discovered the same thing: **crystals can have amazing effects on your health!**

You are about to find *how*...

In this book you will learn all you need to know about the art of crystal healing. By reading this book you will gain an understanding of the **different shapes of crystals**, **types**, and **how they can be used to heal**.

Today, there are many alternate forms of therapy that are widely available. We are learning to extend beyond science and trying to better our lives through natural means.

One such alternate form of therapy is 'Crystal Therapy'. Crystal therapy is an alternative medical technique that employs crystals to restore balance and bring healing to body and mind

There has always been a sense of mysticism associated with crystals, and in recent times even some skepticism around crystal therapy. However, this hasn't stopped people, both commoners and celebrities alike, from utilizing these crystals to bring luck and prosperity into their lives.

For example, celebrities like Adele, Kate Perry and Miranda Kerr swear by the healing effects of crystals. Adele explained how she performed one of her best shows while holding crystals in her hand. And Miranda Kerr even admitted to sleep with her crystals nearby, in order to constantly receive their special healing energies.

We, as a race, have a liking for stones and crystals. The usage of amulets and charms dates back to prehistoric times, though we are not sure of how far back it actually dates. Even today, there are various individuals who have benefited from the healing properties of crystals.

In this book you will be educated about the **basics of crystals** and **how they can be used for healing**. Through this book, I aim to provide you with all the information you require to improve the various aspects of your life.

When you start utilizing the healing crystals, you will find yourself on a journey of **self-discovery** and **exploration**. One that is **serene** and **peaceful**. A **path of growth** - both physically and spiritually.

Let's embark on this journey of discovery and truth together. So make yourself a cup of delicious coffee or tea, sit back, relax and enjoy this magical trip!

1. What Are Crystals?

Key Takeaway: *To understand how crystals can be used for healing, you first need to understand why crystals are so remarkable. Crystals are unique in that they have an almost perfect periodic molecular arrangement. This differentiates crystals from other solids, like rocks and glass. Crystals come in many different shapes, and can be grouped in a crystal family (structure) and crystal habit (shape). The shape is greatly determined by the structure.*

Before we discuss the unique healing effects of crystals, we need to take one step back: what's so special about crystals? And can't you just use a little rock or a piece of glass instead?

Although I will do my best to keep things simple, things may get a little technical in this chapter. However, please bear with me: if you lay a solid foundation now, you will get so much more out of the rest of this book!

***

Crystallization

A crystal is a solid material that is arranged in a repetitive pattern of ions, atoms and molecules. This almost perfect periodic arrangement is called a lattice, and it is what differentiates crystals from other solids such as rocks, metals and glass.

The word crystal derives from word 'krustallos', an Ancient Greek word that can be translated as either 'rock crystal' or simply 'ice'.

Crystals are formed through a process called crystallization. The branch of science dedicated to the study of crystals is known as "crystallography".

Crystals form naturally, in the right conditions. They start out as hot liquids and gasses. The process of crystallization occurs when these liquids and gasses make their way to the earth's surface and start to cool off. This is when they take on their unique shape.

***

Crystals are Different from Rocks and Glass

Crystals have a completely different structure from regular rocks and glass. A collection of atoms is called a unit cell. Unlike rocks and glass, the unit cell in a crystal is repeated over and over again in the same pattern throughout the structure. Due to this arrangement of the atoms, crystals come in peculiar and interesting shapes and colors. Crystals may also have other crystals inside them, and even have other minerals growing inside them.

Each crystal has a different chemical composition, depending upon the minerals and metals that have frozen inside it over time. These minerals that are found in the crystals are what provide them with a "vibration". The healing properties of the crystal depend upon the vibration and composition of the crystal.

***

Crystals Come in Many Different Shapes

Crystals come in a variety of shapes.

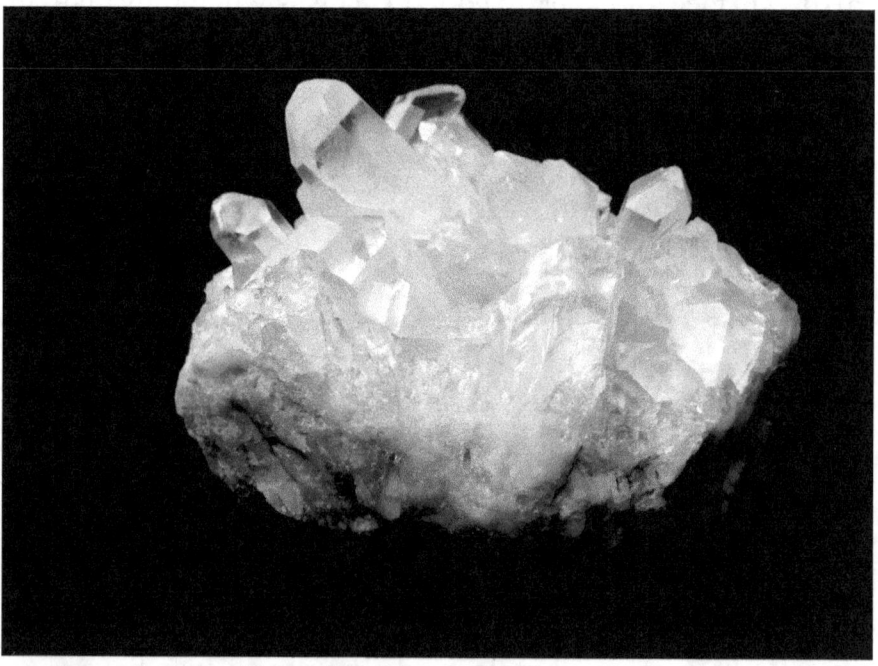

Which form a crystal takes on depends on many factors, such as the temperature and pressure around the time of crystallization. The shape is mostly determined by the crystal structure though.

In order to get a good understanding of the many crystal variations are available, we need to differentiate between a:

- Crystal's structure, referred to as **crystal family**
- Crystal's shape, referred to as **crystal habit**

***

Crystal Families

The crystal structure cannot be seen with the naked eye. It describes in which order the atoms, ions or molecules in a crystal are arranged.

These structures are part of the so called crystal family, which has six members:

- Triclinic
- Monoclinic
- Orthorhombic
- Tetragonal
- Hexagonal (two options here: trigonal and hexagonal)
- Cubic

***

Crystal Habits

The crystal habit on the other hand describes its visible, outward shape. The shape and size of each type of crystal depends upon their internal symmetry and their geometric arrangement. There are many more crystal habits, close to forty.

Here are a few:

- **Acicular** - These crystals have a needle like shape. They are slender and long, but taper towards the ends.
- **Columnar** – These crystals are slender, have prisms that are straight and they are found parallel to each other.
- **Bladed** – These crystals look like blades, hence the name. They are slender and flat crystals.
- **Prismatic** – These crystals are lengthened and are organized as big chunks. They are long structures that resemble a prism.
- **Reniform or coliform** – These crystals are intersecting chunks. They resemble the shape of kidneys.
- **Stubby** – These crystals are wide chunks of rock which are slightly elongated. They have a stubby appearance.
- **Globular** – These crystals are organized as chunks of hemispherical masses which look similar to grapes.

***

Crystal Clusters

Crystals that have grown together in a group are called crystal clusters. These clusters emit energy into the room they are placed in. Additionally, they absorb the negative energy from the room and help in maintaining the balance of the atmosphere in that particular area. As such, they are believed to be superior than regular crystals in enriching the surrounding environment.

These crystals can also be used to bring calmness to a stressful environment like a workplace. They are even given to students to improve their level of concentration.

***

Tumble Stones

When two crystals constantly rub against each other or tumble over each other, the friction that is created between them makes their surfaces smooth and shiny. These smooth and lustrous stones join together and form tumble stones. As a result of these tumbles stones, a balance of energy is created in the person carrying it and this person, in turn, balances the energy of the stone.

***

Cut Crystals

Cut crystals are not naturally found in the environment. Instead, they are formed by cutting and polishing natural crystals. The unique geometry of crystals is the reason behind their positive vibration and healing effects. So if these crystals are cut in the right shape, then the vibration resulting from their geometry will magnify their healing abilities even further.

***

Now you understand the unique properties of crystals. This is just the first step though. The remarkable molecular structure of crystals does not only leave geologists in awe. The reach of crystals is much greater. Crystals have the power to help alleviate physical ailments, bring balance and heal all levels of your being: physical, mental, emotional and spiritual. A wisdom that was shared by ancient civilizations worldwide, across time.

2. What is Crystal Healing

Key Takeaway: *Crystals have been used since the beginning of time. Crystals have always been thought to possess a power that a person cannot completely comprehend or think of logically. Crystals have been known to possess many properties like healing, being a lucky charm, and bringing wealth and prosperity. Crystal healing, also known as crystal therapy, is a medical practice in which crystals are used to cure the ailments of the body and mind. These crystals also serve to protect the body and mind from further diseases that might occur. Adherents of this technique believe that this is an effective treatment strategy.*

In crystal healing, crystals act as conductors during the healing process. These crystals allow the positive, healing energy to flow into the body and they expel or remove the negative, illness causing energy.

This technique of crystal healing has gained popularity since the latter decades of the 20th century. As you just learned, crystals possess a strong geometric structure. This unique property is the reason that they have healing powers. Each kind of crystal has an atomic structure that is unique to it. The unique resonance of each type of crystal is a result of this unique structural arrangement and this resonance is the reason why these crystals possess healing properties.

To use them for healing, the crystals are placed on and around the body. These crystals can either be:

- placed at particular points on the body, or
- spread over the body in a distinct manner that will help to eliminate the negative energy from the body and bring relief.

***

Crystal Healing Throughout the Ages

Although this method has become extremely popular in the last few decades, ancient records have shown us that the technique of crystal healing dates back to more than 6000 years.

Sumerians and Egyptians possess the oldest records of utilizing crystals to help the body heal and to bring balance back to the body. These crystals have also been used by other ancient civilizations like ancient Indian tribes in North-America, Mayans, and Hawaiians. Moreover, in the eastern tradition crystals played a prominent role in relation to balancing the chakras. And the Chinese were particularly in love with the jade crystal, which they believed had a healing effect on the kidney.

Sure, there are some skeptics out there who refer to crystals as pseudoscience. But isn't it striking that all these civilizations, seemed to believe that these crystals had powers associated with them? Remember: these are the times before globalization and internet. Nowadays, by simply opening your browser you have access to more information than Bill Clinton had when he was president of the United States. Only 20 years ago! But the Mayans had no idea about the Chinese or Egyptian culture and their traditions. Yet all these cultures cherished the crystals for their healing powers. Coincidence?

***

Healing Through Resonance

Crystals emit a unique energy vibration. Through the process of resonance, these crystals can be used for a wide variety of purposes. They help bring about a balance of energy in our bodies and, as a result, speed up the body's healing mechanism.

Just like people differ from one another, so do these crystals. This is the reason why the vibration of crystals will guide different kinds of people towards different kinds of crystals.

The body's capacity to resonate with a crystal is dependent upon the state of the body and the mind of the particular individual at that given moment. Every person is connected to his or her own crystal and most people will be able to feel this connection soon after they come in contact with their crystal.

***

Crystals and the Human Body

Every living organism vibrates at a certain frequency or range that is specific to them. These vibrations are the result of the electromagnetic waves present in the living system. These waves possess a specific path. For example, migratory birds resonate with the electromagnetic waves of the earth to discover the right paths across oceans and continents without getting lost.

Humans are also vibrate with electromagnetic waves. However, in us humans the electromagnetic wave system is a little more complex than the system present in other organisms.

Crystals are found to be natural conductors of electromagnetic waves. They have the capacity to help conduct these waves in a balanced manner throughout our bodies. The electromagnetic waves present in our bodies do not follow a random pattern; rather, they seem to possess certain energy centers where they are concentrated. Crystals possess the capacity to activate these centers of energy and this soothes our mind and body, by allowing positive energy to flow through our body. This way, crystals can help balance the negative flow of energy in our bodies and heal all kinds of ailments, whether it is at the physical, emotional, mental or spiritual level of our being.

***

Metaphysical Properties of Crystals

Every crystal possesses its own metaphysical properties. It is as a result of these properties that the crystals have a positive effect on the body. When you use these crystals you will feel a soothing and calming effect spreading throughout your body.

Mentioned below are some properties that explain the healing effects of crystals:

- **Crystals have the power to provide you with braveness and strength**. You will feel powerful and you will feel like you possess the power to rise up to any situation and defend yourself, if required.
- **Crystals are also known to reenergize your body at all four levels – physical, mental, emotional and spiritual**. As a result, it helps creativity flow through your body.
- **The working of crystals adheres to the "Yin and Yang theory"**. This theory is very famous in the Chinese culture, as they believe that every object that exists in the universe is made of two forces that resist and oppose each other. The Yin is the force that represents femininity, while the Yang depicts masculinity. The crystal will help to balance these forces in your body. The energy that is produced from the clashing of these two forces is absorbed by the crystals and thus, leaves you feeling empowered.
- **Crystals usually help to purify your mind and body**. In addition to this, you will be able to balance

the energy in your body by adjusting all the levels of energy in your body collectively.
- **Healing crystals always help to clear your third eye chakra**. While you are meditating, these crystals can help you focus better. It is recommended that you hold a crystal in your hand while meditating.
- **It has been seen that crystals have a great impact on the concentrating and focusing ability of the brain**. These crystals are a boon for students and they love to use some of the crystals that have been mentioned in the chapters that follow as they help them avoid distraction. As a result, they witness an increase in their examination scores. Working professionals are also advised to put these crystals to use, as they will help them improve their working abilities.
- **The crystals are the mirrors to your soul as they can connect your physical body to the astral body**. You will be able to observe every inch of your soul when you use crystals to heal you and you will also be able to obtain the energies of these astral bodies to heal and balance your body.

***

These are the main properties of crystals. Next up, we will get more specific on how you can use crystals for the purpose of healing.

3. Crystal Healing 101

Key Takeaway: *Crystals have the power to transform one form of energy into another. In crystal healing therapy, the energy in these crystals blends with the energy in your body to purify body and mind. Crystal therapy is completely safe, as long as you work under the guidance of a qualified healer. Never solely rely on crystal therapy for healing. If you have a serious illness or physical ailment, please consult your physician.*

You may be pondering about how a tiny piece of rock can actually help you heal. Is that possible, how does it work? Don't worry; in this chapter I will try to answer all your questions. There is a basis behind the working of crystal therapy. Crystal therapy has been successful for many individuals and has made them both physically and mentally healthy.

Let's begin by taking a closer at the healing properties of crystals.

***

Healing Properties of Crystals

These crystals are stones that have been present on Earth since the beginning of time. Crystals are used in the healing of physical, emotional, spiritual and mental ailments. There may be times when you may possess a crystal that has been passed down for several generations. For all you know, this crystal may even be millions of years old. The fun fact here is that you could be utilizing a crystal that was formed a million years ago - it may even date back to the time of the dinosaurs!

The science of metaphysics claims that crystals can transform us. The toughest part of crystal healing is discovering which crystals have healing properties. The healer usually knows how to identify these crystals. For instance, white stones are used in the healing of spiritual problems.

All the stones and crystals that are used for healing work in different ways. Some of the larger stones can also be utilized to cleanse the crystals. Wand-shaped crystals have found extensive use in meditation and healing specific to a particular organ.

***

Crystals Are Energetically Charged

It may come as a surprise, but you should know that all crystals are electrically charged. Crystals are stones that are strong, solid and always organized extremely well. The structure of your crystal rarely changes, regardless of the outside temperature or any other external factor. It doesn't matter how hot it is outside, your crystal remains unaffected by all this. The fact is that these crystals are even capable of surviving global warming.

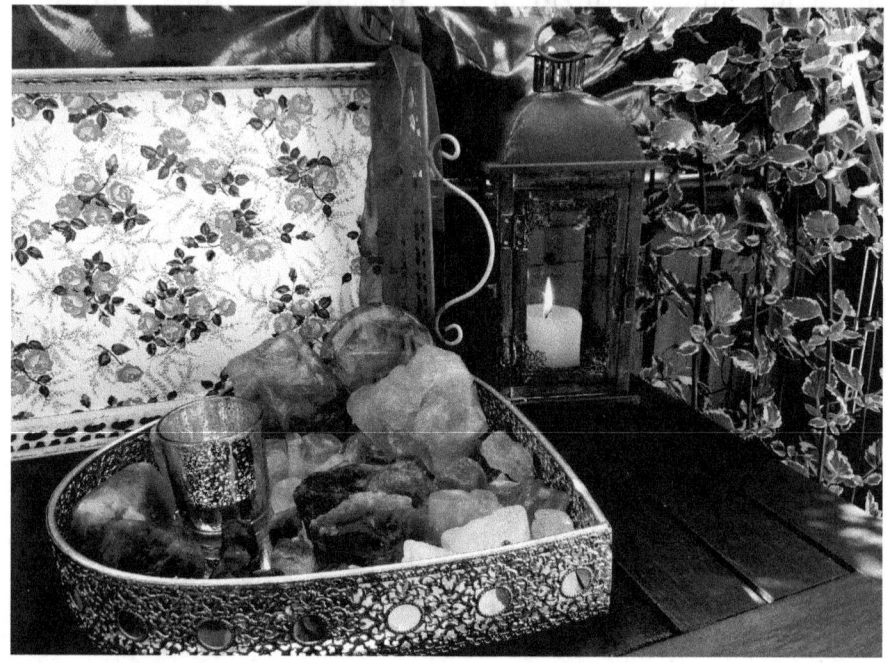

Extra electrons are stored within the lattices of the crystals. It is as a result of these electrons that crystals are able to transform one form of energy into another. When a crystal is either subjected to pressure or heated, it changes its form and converts itself into another stone. This energy can be utilized to heal a person.

The basic essence of every human is energy. Each crystal has its own unique energy that has been stored deep within the heart of the crystal. When crystals are utilized for healing, the energy emanating from the crystal blends with the energy emanating from a person's body, and thus intensifies the energy within the body. In this way it helps in re-balancing the energy within the body. These crystals have the power to change the way we think in ways one cannot begin to fathom.

As the energy from the crystal is utilized to heal a person's body, it is better if the crystal is modified to suit the needs of the person.

The major reason why these crystals have a positive and calming impact on our bodies is because of the metaphysical properties associated with them.

Crystals help to re energize our bodies at the physical, emotional, spiritual and mental levels. They rightly orient these four energy levels and help maintain a balance among them. In short: crystals purify body and mind.

They also assist in maintaining the balance between the Yin and Yang. Yin and Yang are considered to be opposing forces - the Yin is the feminine force, while the Yang is the masculine force. By stabilizing these two forces, the crystals maintain the balance in our aura.

Crystals help to improve one's concentration and clear the third eye while meditating. Moreover, crystals help increasing intuitive prowess of an individual. In addition to all this, they are also utilized to improve a person's communication skills and instill strength and confidence in them.

How Does Crystal Healing Therapy Work

During your research of alternative therapies, you may have come across a plethora of treatment methods that sparked your interest. Perhaps you even tried some of those different methods and techniques that aim to help you heal; both physically and spiritually.

However, let me tell you, of all the techniques that you may have come across, crystal healing is certainly the best and easiest!

Crystal healing is alternatively known as crystal therapy. This method of healing is inexpensive and causes no harm to your body. As you already know, the healing process works only with the energy that is already present in your body. The energy that is present in these crystals blends with the energy that is in your body and either increases or decreases the amount of energy in your body in order to create a balance. At the end of this healing process you will feel refreshed and rejuvenated. The four different levels that exist within you – physical, mental, spiritual and emotional, will be well balanced.

You must always remember that the crystal you pick for yourself is the one that you are most adjusted to. You will discover that this crystal works wonders when you are using it to heal yourself. This is because the crystal is in tune with your spiritual and physical energies and this, in turn will help you heal better.

Working with crystals is simple and easy! All you are required to do is stand around the crystals and let the energy of the crystal work its magic on you. There are various techniques you can utilize to heal and cleanse yourself. The chapters that follow will help you understand these techniques better. The easiest way to heal yourself with the help of a crystal is by simply holding it in your hand!

You should remember to cleanse your crystals regularly, which we will discuss in more detail later on. As the crystal absorbs the energy from your body, it stores that energy within itself. The fact is that the crystal cannot differentiate between positive and negative energy. As a result of this the used crystals tend to have a buildup of energy within them and this energy begins to obstruct the healing properties associated with the crystals. Before you use the crystals in healing, you will be required to cleanse the crystal, which we will get to in a moment. A cleansed crystal heals better than a dirty one. Once you cleanse it you will be able to remove any lingering energy within the crystal and, as a result, you will restore all of its healing powers.

***

Is Crystal Therapy Safe?

Crystals and their healing properties often mesmerize people. Even though there is something truly magical and transformational about crystal healing, a lot of people have doubts about its safety. I would like to clear those doubts. Crystal healing is safe and effective. The concept of crystal healing dates back to prehistoric times. During this time, people made use of crystals for checking the climate, healing physical and mental ailments and so much more.

Even though crystal healing has effective healing properties, it should not be used in the place of conventional medicines. Rather, it should be used in addition to conventional treatment methods for better healing. Crystal healing does not give rise to any side effects, nor does it influence a person's religious beliefs. On the contrary, it is actually based on strong scientific principles with the sole intention of improving the health of mankind. It has been found that after a crystal healing session, most patients reported to have experienced a sense of wellbeing and calm. This shift in mood has been proven to be effective in healing a person.

However, you need to remember that crystal healing needs to be done by an expert practitioner. You need to make sure that your crystal healer is credible and knowledgeable before starting the process of healing. Always make sure to look for a healer who is well experienced and don't start the process of healing till you are completely convinced of their expertise. The mind has a very big role to play in crystal healing. Do not let the practitioner pressure you into getting treatments that you are not comfortable with. In addition to this, make sure that they adhere to strict hygiene and safety standards.

One of the most commonly asked questions about crystal healing is about whether it is safe to be done on people of all age groups. Crystals possess powerful properties, but are completely safe and can be used by everyone.

Crystal healers, who perform the healing, are well qualified professionals. Although there are no licensed crystal healing practitioners currently, they get trained by competent professionals. This gives them in depth knowledge about the working of crystals, which type of crystals are to be used for varied purposes, how to perform the healing, etc.

Some crystal healers work along with general physicians and help them by providing relaxation therapies. However, those who are looking for an expert healer should directly contact the crystal healing association. All in all, crystal healing has been found to have no obvious side effects and is a safe treatment option for everyone.

***

These are the basics of crystal healing. Before we get more specific and discuss the different types of crystals, how to buy, use and cleanse them, let's first discuss another key characteristic of crystals: how they are connected to the chakras.

4. Crystals And Their Connection To The Chakras

Key Takeaway*: Eastern philosophy teaches us that every human being has multiple bodies. Not only a physical body, but also an energy, emotional, mental and spiritual body. The energy body has 7 main chakras. If you have practiced yoga, you may already be familiar with the chakras. The word chakra is Sanskrit and translates as wheel. So chakras are wheels of energy. Balanced chakras have a positive effect on the other bodies. If there is an imbalance in one of your chakras, this may result in symptoms in other bodies: physical ailments, feeling negative emotions, etc. Crystals can help restore balance in the chakras. By understanding the effect that crystals have upon your chakras you can use them to your benefit.*

The existence of chakras are a key element in the Eastern tradition, especially in Tantra Yoga and Tibetan Buddhism. The word chakra comes from Sanskrit, and translates as wheel. Chakras are wheels of energy that reside in your energy body. We have multiple bodies. Not only the physical body, that can be seen with the naked eye, but also an energy, emotional, mental and spiritual body.

Why are we talking about chakras in a book about crystal healing?

***

Laws of Correspondence and Resonance

According to this Eastern philosophy, there are two important universal laws that everyone is bound by:

- **The law of correspondence**
- **The law of resonance**

The **law of correspondence** teaches that the essence of whatever is out there in the universe is also found in a human being, and vice versa. Not literally of course, you won't find a giant tree inside you. But the essence of everything. For example, the sun gives off heat. In our body there is also something that regulates our body temperature, to maintain homeostasis. You could call this your inner sun.

The **law of resonance** teaches that everything in existence has a vibrational frequency, with which it is possible to resonate. As an illustration, think of two identical tuning forks. Striking one tuning fork will cause the other to resonate at the same frequency. A tuning fork that rings at a different vibrational frequency will not resonate with the original tuning fork. According to the law of resonance, you can amplify a vibrational frequency within you by resonating with its universal counterpart outside you. So for example: if you are always cold, you can use techniques that will allow you to tune into and resonate with the vibrational frequency of universal heat.

***

How These Laws Connect to the Chakras

Your chakras are your antennas, your tools of resonance. A human being has seven chakras, most of them are located just in front of the body and connect to the spine. So contrary to what you may find in some popular new age books, chakras are not located in the physical body. They are connected to the physical body, but are actually located in the energy body, just outside the physical body.

The lowest, first chakra is located at the level of your perineum, and the seventh chakra is located above your head. The others are in between these two, in front of the body.

Each chakra governs different aspects of our life. Take the first or root chakra for example; this chakra is related to vitality, survival and feeling safe. Are you often experiencing feelings of fear, without good reason (you are not in a life-threatening situation)? If so, that is an indication that you have an imbalance in your root chakra.

The law of correspondence teaches us that whatever is in you is also out there. This means you can increase your feeling of safety by resonating with the vibrational frequency of safety out there in the universe. An excellent way to do this is the use of crystals.

***

Crystals and Their Effect on Chakras

Crystals help in cleansing and energizing your chakras and your energy. In order to heal successfully, these crystals need to be placed on the focus points of the chakras.

When they are placed in this manner, their vibrating energy will balance the flow of energy in your body and cleanse it. Once the energy flowing in your body is cleansed, your body automatically syncs and becomes in harmony with the positive energy. This helps the healing process.

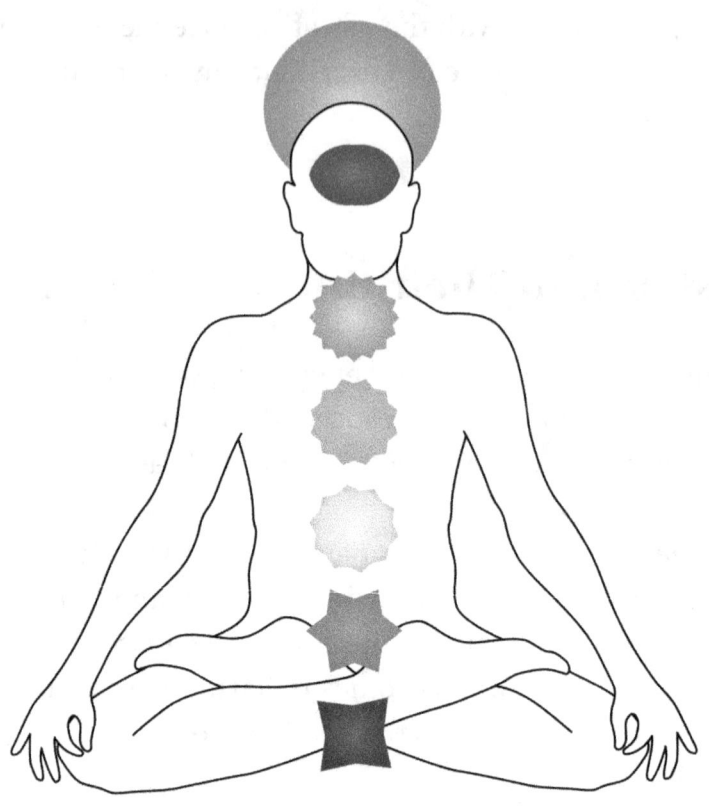

There are seven main chakras:

1. **Root (Muladhara)**
2. **Sacral (Svadisthana)**
3. **Navel (Manipura)**
4. **Heart (Anahata)**
5. **Throat (Vishuddha)**
6. **Third Eye / Middle of Forehead (Ajna)**
7. **Crown (Sahasrara)**

When the crystal-healing technique is used, these seven points need to be focused upon.

Let's take a closer look at each chakra.

***

The Root Chakra – Muladhara

This chakra is situated just below the genitals, at the perineum, below the base of the spine. It governs our sense of safety and security. In this life, we strive to accomplish our goals, be it business or materialistic. It is this chakra that gives us the power to attain these goals.

If a feeling of exasperation, insecurity, uneasiness or fearfulness lingers around you, it is likely because of the obstruction of the root chakra's energy flow. At a physical level, the root chakra is associated with the hips, legs and lower back.

To purify this chakra, use crystals that are brown, red or black in color.

***

The Sacral Chakra – Svadisthana

This chakra is located about two - three inches above the genitals. This chakra is the core of your basic needs for sexuality, imagination, creativity, instinctiveness and self-worth.

It also controls the level of confidence and self-worth and your capability to socialize.

When your emotions move easily, without any disruption, then there is a proper stability in your sacral chakra. The sexual organs are associated with this chakra.

To purify this chakra, use crystals that are mainly orange in color.

***

The Navel Chakra - Manipura

This chakra is positioned in front of the navel (and not the solar plexus, a common misconception).

Manipura chakra is the source of personal strength, self-esteem, warrior energy and power of transformation. Self-confidence, sense of purpose, courage, honour and sense of motivation are a result of this chakra. If one lacks these aspects, then their chakra is out of balance.

The body parts associated with this chakra are the stomach, liver, gallbladder, pancreas and the small intestine.

To purify this chakra, use crystals that are primarily brown in color.

***

The Heart Chakra – Anahata

This chakra is located in front of the heart.

It is the core of unconditional love and compassion. It is centered between 3 lower and 3 higher chakras, and as such beautifully showcases that love is the gateway to connect the earthly realm with the spiritual realm.

A balanced heart chakra results in feelings of compassion, friendliness, empathy and a need to nurture others unconditionally. Conversely, an imbalanced heart chakra is likely to lead to feelings of selfishness, self-pity, indecisiveness, inability to let go and feelings of being unworthy of love. This chakra is associated with the heart, circulatory system, lungs, upper back and shoulders.

To purify this chakra, use crystals that are mainly green and pink in color.

***

The Throat Chakra – Vishuddha

This chakra is located in front of the throat, at the lower part of the neck, in the area that looks like a V of your collarbone.

Vishuddha chakra works as the focal point of your communication, sound and the capacity to express your creativity through your thoughts, your capacity to write and your speech. The other areas that the throat chakra controls are your possibilities for transformation, change and healing.

If you feel that you usually hold back, if you are shy and you prefer to keep quiet, if you seem to feel weak or if you have difficulty in expressing your thoughts then it usually is a sign that means that this chakra is imbalanced.

However, if you feel balanced, centered, and you have a bout of musical or artistic inspiration and you usually are a good speaker, then it signifies that this chakra is in balance with your mind and body; and that the flow of energy is not blocked.

To purify this chakra, use crystals that are light blue in color.

***

The Third Eye Chakra - Ajna

The sixth chakra is known as the Third Eye and is located in front of the middle of your forehead.

The third eye usually serves as the focal point for any psychic ability you might possess, your higher intuition and your energies of light and spirit. It also governs any type of telepathy or astral travel, memories of past lives, as well as your capability to focus and concentrate.

If you feel that you are not assertive, if you have the fear of not succeeding, or if you choose to go the other way and be egotistical, then it is an indication that your third eye chakra is imbalanced.

When you choose to stand up and decide that you can live your life without fearing death, if you are not materialistic, that is a sign that your third eye is perfectly balanced, it is open and the energy is smoothly flowing through the center.

To purify this chakra, use crystals that are dark blue or purple in color.

***

The Crown Chakra - Sahasrara

The seventh chakra is located at the top of your head, just above the fontanel.

This chakra serves as the focal point of your spirituality, your productive thoughts, your enlightenment and your energy. The crown or the seventh chakra, when not blocked, allows an inward flow of spiritual wisdom.

If you are constantly frustrated, only focused on life on earth, or if you don't seem to enjoy life or have the zest for it and if you have negative feelings or thoughts, that is a sign that this chakra is not in balance with your mind and your body. When this chakra is imbalanced, you may start to feel sick and these illnesses could include migraine headaches or you might feel depressed.

To purify this chakra, use crystals that are white or purple in color.

***

You now have a good understanding of the unique properties that crystals have, and how their healing powers can bring balance to body and mind. Are you getting excited about trying it out for yourself? I am sure you are getting more and more enthusiastic to get your hands on some crystals and do your own experiment!

The earth has blessed us with a great variety in crystals. But that variety can also be somewhat overwhelming! So let's take a look at the many different crystals that are available to you, so you can make an informed decision once you feel drawn to a particular crystal.

5. Eight Essential Healing Crystals

Key Takeaway: *In your journey towards discovering the powers of crystals, you will come across a wide variety of crystals. Don't go crystal shopping without reading up on the different types of crystals beforehand, or you will likely be disappointed. In this chapter we will take a look at some of the most popular and powerful crystals.*

This chapter will help you find those crystals and understand their properties in detail. Once you are done with this chapter, you will have a lot more clarity regarding crystals!

It is impossible to discuss every crystal out there in this book. But below you will find some of the most powerful ones. You can't really go wrong with any of these.

These are the crystals that we will examine more closely:

1. Clear Quartz
2. Rose Quartz
3. Citrine
4. Amethyst
5. Hematite
6. Fluorite

7. Black Tourmaline
8. Amazonite

***

Clear Quartz

A clear quartz is the best possible crystal available for healing. This crystal has no negative side effects. The only thing you need to keep in mind is that it needs to be thoroughly cleansed after each use.

You will be able to balance the different energies in your body – physical, mental, spiritual and emotional, by using the clear quartz crystal. You will have the capacity to align all the energies in your body. It is very easy to cleanse this crystal and you will discover that it is easy to program the crystal that will help you balance all the energies in your body. This crystal will create a great impression on your soul.

***

Rose Quartz

The rose quartz crystal is one that represents every aspect of love. This crystal works best for the heart (Anahata) chakra.

You will be able to get a better understanding of the way your heart works and you will have the capacity to comprehend your feelings. This crystal will also help in increasing your faith and trust in the people around you. You will learn to unconditionally love yourself and this, in turn, will help in introducing you to your inner self. Moreover, using this crystal will remove any feelings of grief and depression.

Once you learn to love yourself, you will be able to overcome any negative thoughts you may have about yourself. Any feelings of resentment that you have towards the people around you will vanish once you start using this crystal.

***

Citrine

Citrine is often referred to as the abundance stone. You will find that you are filled with joy and warmth after using this stone.

The energy you have when you use this crystal is out of the world! You will start believing in yourself and will also be able to stimulate the forces of the mind that would help you communicate with your inner self. It always gives you everything you need in abundance; wealth, happiness, self-confidence and so on!

***

Amethyst

This crystal has the ability to convert all the negative energy in your body to positive energy.

You will be able to access your subconscious when you use this crystal, as well as access a meditative state during the healing process. It is because of this that you can even use amethyst to balance your third eye chakra!

The stone is extremely spiritual and helps you access the higher self. This crystal, like the clear quartz, is very good for spiritual healing; it allows you to transform and heal yourself.

***

Hematite

Hematite is the perfect friend for your mind.

This crystal works towards purging your mind from any negative thoughts. These thoughts are terrible for you since they bring you down mentally and emotionally. Your mind will begin to open itself up and start observing the world around you more.

The advantage of this crystal is that you will be able to remove any inhibitions you may have with respect to the different aspects in your life. If you use this crystal along with clear quartz, you will be able to regain the balance of your mind. Finally, using this crystal also cleanses your blood.

***

Fluorite

Fluorite helps you balance your thoughts and also help your mind focus more on the task you have at hand.

This crystal helps in stabilizing any influence that you may have on you at any level. For example, when you talk to somebody you will find that you have a higher sense of understanding.

***

Black Tourmaline

The black tourmaline crystal is called the protection stone because it creates a protective shield around your body and your mind to ward off any negativity.

Using it will enable you to remove any amount of fear you may feel. Moreover, you will be able to enhance your inspiration and learn on your own. This crystal will greatly boost your confidence!

***

Amazonite

The Amazonite crystal is another delight!

It helps in creating balance between your physical body and the astral (mental) body. It also helps in aligning your body's energy levels. Amazonite helps in calming you down and enhances your creativity by increasing your power of imagination.

***

These are some of the most beneficial crystals that you can use. Time to get your first crystals! Let's hop online, go to Amazon and...

Hold it right there.

Buying the right crystal is not the same as buying coffee beans. Remember what we discussed about how many people feel pulled towards a particular crystal? This happens greatly on your current state and energy balance. It may almost feel as if the crystal chooses you.

So what is the best place to buy crystals: in a shop, or online? That's what we will discuss next.

6. Buying Crystals: Online or in a Store?

Key Takeaway: *Now that you have acquired knowledge about the different type of crystals, the next step is to buy them. Are you wondering about how to do that? Purchasing crystals can be tricky but we are here to help you understand which is the right buy for you.*

More and more, consumers are shifting towards buying goods online. It's just so convenient, right? Amazon reported a staggering 2016 sales revenue of $135.99 billion, up from $107.01 billion in 2015!

With every product you want just a finger click away, it may be tempting to just order your crystals online. But is this the best way to go about buying your crystals?

Choosing the right crystal(s) is a delicate matter. Why? Because which crystal you will feel drawn to greatly depends on what's happening within you right now. Touching different crystals, and holding them in your hands, will greatly increase your chances of finding the perfect match. Keep this in mind when shopping online.

***

Buying a Crystal in a Store

When you are shopping for crystals, it is not necessary to know every single detail of every crystal you are considering to buy. All that you are required to do is to have an open mind. By doing this, your mind and body will help direct you to the crystal that best suits your needs. Each person has a special connection to his or her crystal and you will be able to sense this connection when you are purchasing your crystal.

There may be circumstances where you may feel confused about which crystal you need to buy, but worrying or stressing at this time will be of no help. Here's a tip: lay the selection of crystals in front of you, close your eyes and take in slow deep breaths until your body and mind are relaxed and calm. Once your mind and body become calm, the choice will be clearer and you will now know which crystal is the right choice for you. Now, slowly open your eyes while in that state of calmness and pick the crystal you feel most connected to and in sync with.

***

Buying a Crystal Online

Some of you may not have the time or be in the right circumstances to go and purchase a crystal in a shop. In such case, you could use the Internet and purchase them online.

If you are hinging towards an online purchase, remember that this not allow you to touch the crystals, and get a feel for it. During times like these, it is best to trust your intuitions. But, if you still feel confused and are unable to choose from an assortment of different crystals, then it is better not to make a purchase, as it may not be the right time for you yet.

Your mind and your brain are not the same thing. Your brain is the central organ of your body, while your mind is the mental state of both your body and spirit. To make this simple, you could say that the mind of every person has two distinct 'places'. The first place is your conscious mind; which is your active mental state in which you are aware of what is happening around you and this is the part of your mind that panics and stresses and is constantly working. The other part is your subconscious mind; this part is always calm and it is the place that knows your innermost thoughts and desires.

Your conscious mind may be in a constant state of change and it usually does not know what crystal works best for you. But, your subconscious is always calm and your thoughts and desires are fixed in it. So it is really important that you get in touch with your sub-conscious while selecting your healing crystal and the only way to do this is by calming yourself and your conscious mind. This way you will not be confused or have any doubts when you are purchasing your crystal and you will be able to make the right choice.

If you order a crystal online, make sure you order with a company that allows you to return the crystals at no additional cost within a certain period of time. This way you won't lose any money if you open the package and immediately sense that, although these crystals look beautiful, you don't feel any energetic connection to them.

***

Other than your intuition, what is the best way to go about selecting the right crystals to work with? That's what we will cover in the next chapter.

7. Five Tips to Ensure You Get the Most Out of Your Crystals

Key Takeaway: To get the most out of your crystals, it is important to do your research and get a feel for them before buying them. Once you have bought your crystal, program and cleanse them regularly. Also experiment with different ways of using the crystals.

Even if you intend to buy your crystals online, I still recommend you first visit a crystal shop first and get a feel for what's for sale.

To maximize the healing effects of the crystals you work with, here are five tips to ensure you get the most out of your crystals:

1. **Do your research**
2. **Feel the emerging energy from the crystal**
3. **Program your crystals**
4. **Cleanse your crystals**
5. **Experiment with different ways of using the crystals**

***

Tip 1: Do Your Research

It is of extreme importance that you do the required research and gather information as you can. This information should not be just about the healing properties of the crystals, but also the ways in which you can use them. Reading this book is a good starting point. But if you are serious about crystals, make sure to also check other resources.

***

Tip 2: Feel the Emerging Energy from the Crystal

When you are looking to buy healing crystals, it is crucial that you hold the crystal in your hand and try to see how the energy emerging from the stone interacts with your own energy.

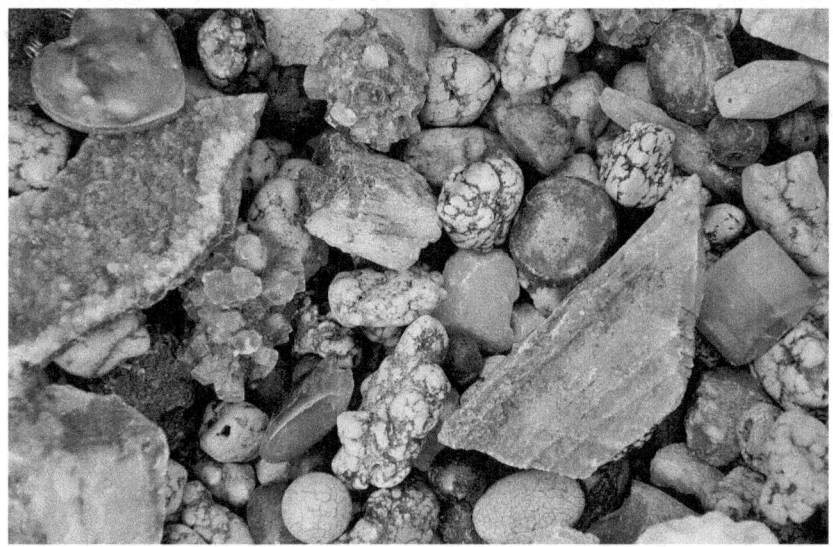

The next thing that you need to do is close your eyes and see if you can feel any slight sensations such as tingling in either your hands or arms. While doing this, remember to pay attention to the sensations in the other parts of your body that might be caused because of the energy from the crystal.

If you are buying a crystal online, you could try to practice this simple step. Retire to a quiet place and close your eyes. While your eyes are closed, visualize the crystal and focus on it. See how the stone makes you feel on a physical, emotional and spiritual level. That will give you a strong indication of whether this crystal is right for you or not.

***

Tip 3: Program your Crystals

Intention plays a very important role while you are utilizing stones, crystals or any other elements of the earth for the purpose of physical, mental, spiritual and emotional healing.

Always remember to program the crystals with your intention. Programing the crystals is easy and simple, all you need to do is place these crystals in your hands and meditate with them.

***

Tip 4: Cleanse the Crystals

If you want your crystals to maintain their resonance for a long period of time, you will need to cleanse your crystals on a regular basis. We will cover how to cleanse your crystals in more detail in chapter '10. Cleansing Your Crystals'.

***

Tip 5: Experiment With Different Ways of Using the Crystals

Different people use their healing crystals in different ways. There is no need use these crystals in a similar manner as everyone else. You can hold these stones in your hands either while praying or meditating. You can also try incorporating these healing crystals into your jewelry. Likewise, when you are trying to align your chakras you can position these stones on or near the chakras and this will help balance your energies.

***

Next up, we will take a closer look at different ways in which you can use crystals.

8. How to Use These Crystals

Key Takeaway: *There are different ways in which you can use crystals for healing. For example, you can wear them on your body, lie down and place them on a specific body part or chakra location, place them under your pillow or even use them when taking a bath! Do your own experiment, and be creative.*

Crystals can be utilized in a wide variety of ways. In the end, the method used just depends on your energy level and your preference. Here are the best ways in which you can use crystals.

***

Wearing Crystals on Your Body

The simplest way to profit from the healing properties of crystals is by wearing them.

Usually, people have no prior knowledge about the healing properties of a crystal; but they instinctively choose a crystal that seems to have a positive and healing effect on them.

Keep in mind that the length of the chain that your crystal pendant is suspended from also influences the effect of your crystal. For instance, if you are wearing your crystal pendant on a choker, it will be very close to the chakra that governs your throat (Vishuddha), and its greatest effects will be felt in the areas governed by that chakra. But, at the same time, it will still give positive energy to the entire body and maintain the balance.

***

Keeping Crystals Under Your Pillow

Keeping certain crystals under your pillow helps in preventing nightmares, relieving stress and curing insomnia. Some crystals, when kept under the pillow, will help in dream recollection. This is especially helpful if you want to have more lucid dreams.

***

Using Crystals When Taking a Bath

Using crystals while taking a bath is also very effective.

In order for it to work, you must place the crystals inside the bathwater or around the tub you bathe in. When you take a bath, you not only clean your body, but you clean your mind too.

After bathing your mind becomes fresh, you feel relaxed and stress free. The stresses, tensions and strains on your mind are also washed along with dirt when you bathe. Even your negative thoughts and emotions go away when you have a good bath. It will soothe your physical self and your mental state, giving you a fresh start.

***

Meditating with Crystals

Crystals have a stable geometric structure that helps them to vibrate. This vibration will impart stillness in your physical body when you meditate and will help you calm your mind.

When you have a problem, it means there is an unresolved issue that your normal thought process could not overcome. At a time like that, you have to realize that in order for you to solve this problem, you have to change the way you usually think. And when you do that, you will see that you will be able to find a solution to you problem quite easily.

Meditation helps to alter your thought process, as you learn how to observe your thoughts and not identify with them. Crystals amplify this process. While meditating, place the crystals that help you to stay calm in front of you, or you can hold them in your hands if you prefer it that way.

***

Making Crystal Essences

Usually an essence is the liquid form of a solid entity or its energy. Similarly, when the energy patterns of crystals are liquefied they are called a crystal essence, or elixir. Though water is the most common substance on earth, it has certain unique properties that are not present in other substances.

One is that is neutral and can take in other energy forms quite easily, like that of crystals. It is these unique properties of water that help make the gem essence very effective.

Gem essence with water is very simple to make; all you have to do is place the crystal stone of your choice in fresh spring water. Now, leave this bowl out at normal room temperature for the duration of about 10 hours without disturbing it. Gem Essence is much more effective than gem water. However, the advantage of gem water is that you can drink it easily without having to worry about any side effects or reactions that you may experience.

While making a gem essence, always keep in mind that even though crystals have healing powers, the minerals in some crystals are toxic to the body. So to be on the safer side, stick to quartz crystals if you do not know what minerals are present in the crystal that you want to use. Or use two containers. A big container for the water. And a small container for the crystals, which is then placed in the big container. This way, the crystals do not come into direct contact with the water.

***

Now that you have learned the most important ways in which crystals can be used, you may wonder: what exactly are the healing powers of these crystals? What can I expect to use them for?

Well, I'm glad you asked! In the next chapter, you will learn all about how crystals can alleviate symptoms of, and even heal, all kinds of physical ailments.

9. Crystal Healing For Specific Conditions

Key Takeaway: *Crystals are very powerful as a means of protection and for healing purposes. Crystal healing has been found to be successful in treating or alleviating various illnesses and problems. In this chapter, you will learn how you use crystals to treat certain physical and emotional conditions yourself.*

How do you use crystals for specific ailments? So far, you have learned that crystals have a wonderful effect on your being as a whole. But what if you suffer from headaches, or a lack of energy? Can crystals help for these health issues?

The answer is: *yes*.

A word of caution though, before we get into the healing benefits of crystals: do not use this practice in the place of contemporary medical treatments. Rather, use it in addition to those treatments. If you are someone who suffers from serious health problems then it is always a good idea to (also) consult your doctor or health practitioner.

With that said, some medications only treat the symptoms and not the root cause, and can also have some very nasty side effects. And even if treatment is effective, the subtle influence of crystals can be really complementary to any such treatment.

You can experience the various benefits of crystals by just placing them in your homes; they could be placed on a shelf, a table or anywhere that you like. 'Gridding' is the process of positioning crystals in critical areas around one's home. 'Gridding' protects and safeguards the people of that home from negative and malicious energies.

To treat a specific ailment, you would do better to place the crystal on the part of the body that needs healing, or on one or more of the positions where the chakras are located. As mentioned earlier, chakras are considered to be energy wheels or nodes. Each chakra is related to a specific organ in the body. This chakra gives the organ the energy to function. They are also related to specific aspects of behavior and development. As we already know, the state of health and balance in a person depends on the energy that flows through the chakras. This balance is very important to lead a healthy life. Each chakra is an important part of our energy balance.

Now let's see how the use of crystals can help alleviate and even heal health issues like headaches, lack of energy or libido, insomnia, and even finding love.

***

Headaches

A wide variety of crystals can be used to relieve a person from a headache. The crystal to be used depends upon the type of the headache.

Crystals like amber, amethyst or turquoise can be used on the head to relieve tension headache. Lapis lazuli can also be utilized. Amethyst can be placed in a layout that is healing, around the head to drive away the headache.

The imbalance between the head energy and the solar plexus chakra could be source of origin of headaches. Citrine or moonstone can be put to use to cure these headaches by balancing the energy. A headache that arises as a result of stress could also be due to imbalance between solar plexus and head energy.

***

Sleeplessness/Insomnia

Which crystal is best to help cure insomnia depends on what lies at the root of that sleeplessness. You might have to try out various crystals to find out which one works best for you. This is because of the fact that the crystals have different effects for different people.

If stress or tension is the reason that a person suffers from insomnia, then crystals such as rose quartz, chrysoprase, citrine or amethyst can be used to cure this condition. The crystal can either be placed next to the bed or under one's pillow.

If the cause of sleeplessness is overeating, then moonstones or pyrites can be used to help settle one's stomach and help one fall asleep.

Tourmaline or smoky quartz can be utilized if nightmares are the reason for the insomnia. They help one sleep peacefully. They need to be placed at the base of the bed or near the person's feet. Labradorite can also help because it is believed to drive away negative thoughts and feelings.

***

Lack of Energy

Orange, red and yellow crystals help in increasing one's energy. The crystals that are brightly colored are the most zestful ones. Deep red garnets, topaz or golden amber are some varieties of stones that help combat the lack of energy.

To improve motivation, tiger's eye, dark citrine or jasper can be used. Positioning the citrine on the solar plexus and holding clear quartz in both hands in an upward manner results in boosting of one's energy.

***

Lack of Libido

The absence of sexual feelings could be because of negative emotions. If emotions are the reason for the block in sexual energy, red garnets and fluorite can help release them. They help in stimulating the libido once again.

***

Blood Circulation Disorders

Disorders that are connected to the flow of blood such as kidney problems, premenstrual problems or even other problems of the internal organs that are related to the flow of blood can be treated with the aid of certain crystals.

The ancient Chinese medicine tradition considered jade to have particularly healing effect on the kidney. But a lot of crystals are believed to possess the capacity to remove toxins from one's body and improve overall health. This particular property of crystals helps to treat physical problems related to blood flow.

***

Difficulty with Studying and Concentration

Concentration and focus can be enhanced by using quartz. Quartz helps to clear the mind. Carnelian helps remove unnecessary thoughts from the mind. Amber and citrine can be utilized to stimulate memory. Lapis lazuli can be used to amplify thoughts.

When used together they can enhance concentration. When used along with amethyst, these crystals can help a person focus on realistic goals and help their channel their energy towards achieving their goals. They also help to soothe the nervous system.

Fluorite helps one study better. It balances the right and left hemisphere of the brain. When used along with sodalite it helps in improve the communication between the left and right hemispheres of the brain.

***

Healing the Mind

Crystals are also known to promote peace of mind by removing blocks to emotional expression. The crystals that are used for this purpose need to be kept in contact with the body.

Green is thought to be a color that heals, hence green crystals such as jade are used to reduce mental stress as well as nervous stress. They aid in the focusing of the mind.

Rose quartz and blue lace agate are used as detoxifying agents. They help to cleanse a person's emotions. Opal helps to maintain emotional balance and stability. Amethyst helps in the balancing of hormones and emotions. It reduces confusion and increases control. It also helps to relieve stress and mental problems.

Amber is used as a neutralizer. It balances the negative state of the mind and brings it back to normal. It also aids in balancing all sorts of emotional or endocrine problems.

In addition to these issues, crystals can also be used for a wide variety of disorders. The healing and soothing effect that these crystals possess make us understand that healing does not just occur at the physical level. A certain amount of spiritual and mental healing is also needed to achieve a holistic healthy persona.

***

Crystal Healing and Love

Crystals can also be utilized to bring love into your life as they can be utilized to attract your soulmate. While this isn't magic and your soulmate will not materialize in front of you, it will help you clear your mind and as a result you will be more open to the possibility of finding your soulmate.

When a person desperately craves love and affection, their entire mind is consumed by that idea. This becomes an unhealthy obsession. Ultimately, true love focuses on the other, not on filling a hole in oneself.

For a person to naturally fall in love, their mind needs to clear. Crystals will help clear the mind. Rather than just satisfying a person's need temporarily, a crystal will help the person find a permanent solution to their need for love. The emotions related to love often overlap and are confused with the emotions of lust and need. Crystals help separate the two and give you clarity.

There are a wide variety of crystals and stones associated with love. Each stone is related to a different quality of love.

The following list gives you an idea about the different kinds of crystals and stones, and what kind of love healing they help in:

- **Amber** is utilized to help in romantic and marital love.
- **Emeralds** are utilized to help the user find passion and romance.
- **Garnets** help the user find romance.
- **Jade** is a stone that is used universally and helps one connect to any type of love.
- **Kunzite** is utilized to heal blocks in unconditional love like the love between a mother and her child.
- **Lapis lazuli** is utilized to help with marital and spiritual problems.
- **Larimar** is a stone that seems to work for attracting a soulmate. It also gives off love and improves communication in relationships.
- **Moonstones** are usually utilized to heal any kind of problem associated with love.
- **Morganite** attracts love into a person's life. It also helps the person to maintain the love and grow it. In

addition to this, Morganite encourages you to have loving thoughts and actions, reduces stress and helps you to appreciate and enjoy your life.

- **Rose quartz** is the most popular type of love stone. It is the stone of unconditional love. It helps a person love themself, increases their sensitivity and makes them more empathetic. It aids in creating harmony and restores trust in the case of broken relationships. For those who have lost love it offers comfort, and to those who have never known love, it offers a new path. It removes negativity and replaces it with hope and trust. It is sometimes very powerful in its healing that it might need an amethyst to be used along with it to cool it down.
- **Ruby** is considered useful in helping with passion and romance.
- **Sardonyx** is another crystal that is utilized to promote love in the body.
- **Selenite** is usually used to restore all kinds of love.
- **Sodalite** helps with self-love.
- **Topaz** signifies true and spiritual love.

These crystals can be utilized in different ways. They can either be placed under the pillow while sleeping to ensure positive thoughts and dreams about the one you love or they can be placed in a location where you want love to flow around. You can use a crystal wand to focus the energy and emotion on your soulmate. Accessories with these stones can be worn at all times to attract love or help in self-love.

***

These are just some ways in which you can use crystals to treat specific physical or emotional issues. For any condition you may be dealing with, keep the following in mind:

- **Do your research**.
- **Follow your intuition** when picking the crystal. It will pull you toward the one(s) you need to receive healing.
- **Program the crystal** before use, by expressing your intended use and desired outcome
- **Place the crystal** on the part of your body that needs healing, or on the position of the chakra that you want to work with.

Regardless of which crystals you use, and what you use them for, you need to take proper care of them. Crystals are neutral of themselves, but if you use them for healing, they will take on some of the negative energy you are trying to get rid off. You wouldn't eat your breakfast from the same plate you used for dinner yesterday without first doing the dishes, right? With crystals, take the same approach.

Next up, you will learn how you can make sure your crystals are always ready for use!

10: Cleansing Your Crystals

***Key Takeaway**: To ensure that your crystals keep on performing optimally during crystal healing therapy, cleanse them regularly. There are different techniques you can use, such as smudging, moonlight clearing and the sacred breath. Experiment with all of them. Program your crystals after the cleansing, and they will be as good as new again!*

There may be times when a crystal that you felt strongly drawn to initially, suddenly does not feel like it is right for you anymore. Somehow, the connection that you had with that crystal feels wrong now.

This is a sign that indicates that your crystal needs cleaning. If your crystals are not properly cleaned before they are used in the healing process, the healing will not take place properly and the crystals will not provide your mind and your body with the results that you seek.

The clearer the energy associated with a healing crystal, the more powerful its effectiveness will be. Even if the crystals are brand new, you must remember to clear your healing crystal after you purchase them. Similarly, you should also remember to clear your healing crystals well after every healing session.

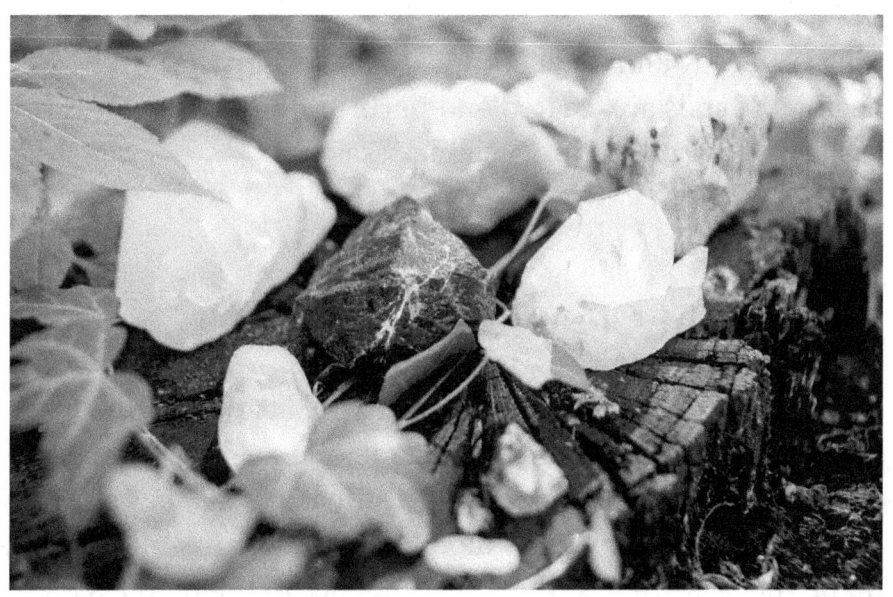

When the clearing of a crystal is done properly, it will feel tingly, bright, positive and cold to touch. If your crystal starts to feel hot, heavy or drained, that is an indication that it needs to be cleansed.

Below you will find the most effective methods to cleanse your crystal.

***

Smudging

This technique is simple and easy to use. All you need to do is to smudge your healing crystal with burning sage or cedar. While smudging, hold the burning cedar stick or sage and gently pass your healing crystal through its smoke.

This is an easy and excellent way to make sure that your healing crystals are cleared and purified. Smudging can easily be done after every healing session.

***

Moonlight Clearing

Moonlight clearing is another effective way to clear your healing crystals. For this cleaning method be sure to choose a full moon night and place all the healing crystals that need to be cleared under the direct moon light. Why a full moon night? Because this is when the influence of the moon is the strongest, which makes it the best time to dispel any negative energy that your crystal could be carrying.

The amount of time that is required to clear your crystals depends upon the sensitivity of the healer. Also, the amount of material that needs to be cleared from your crystals depends upon the person on whom the healing was done.

If you cannot find a suitable flat surface to put your crystals on under the moonlight, tie them to strings and hang them from a tree or any support that faces the moonlight.

The moonlight is gentle and it does not have any heat energy of its own. This is the reason we use moonlight for clearing the healing crystals instead of sunlight. If you place your healing crystals under the sun, they may start to fade and lose their color. Also, as a result of the intensity of the sun's rays, your crystals will get internal fractures, which may cause your crystals to break.

**

Burying

The technique of burying to clear your healing crystals is also quite simple.

All you need to do is bury the healing crystals that have to be cleared in a jar or cup filled with dried herbs. The dried herbs that are usually used for this technique are rose petals, frankincense, myrrh, sage and sandalwood. These ingredients are easily available and they are friendly on the wallet. This technique used for clearing crystals is easy and effective.

However, if you feel that you require a deeper cleansing using this method, bury your healing crystals in the earth. People who own gardens can select a cozy corner in their gardens and people who live in apartments or flats could make use of a good flowerpot. Dig a hole in the soil and place the healing crystals that need to be cleared in them. The size of the hole shouldn't be too big for the crystal. After this is done, cover the crystal with more soil and leave it there. The amount of time you keep your crystals buried is totally up to you. You could mark the place where you buried your crystals so that it will be easier to find them when you wish to remove them.

***

Sacred Breath

The sacred breath technique is does not require a lot of effort or the use of any extra materials. If you want a very simple method to clear your crystals, you can choose this one.

Hold the crystal that needs to be cleared in your hand and gently blow away all the negative and heavy energy that has built up inside it. While engaging in this technique your mind needs to be calm. You should ask your higher self to slowly clean the crystal and clear it of any bad energy it might have.

***

Cool Water

If you are in a hurry and it is a real emergency, but your crystals really need to be cleared NOW, then using water is the fastest way to clear your crystals.

Pour cold water all over your healing crystals. When you are running cold water over your crystals, make sure that the points of the crystal are facing downwards, towards the drain. This will run all of the negative energy present inside your crystals right down your sink.

Just make sure that the water is cold before you start running it over your crystals, because warm water might break or fracture your crystal.

***

Programming Your Crystals After the Cleanse

Once you have bought a new crystal and have cleared it using any of the aforementioned methods, it is a good idea to program – or charge – your crystal again. You have bought that crystal for some specific need or healing; programming your crystal to that particular need will intensify the effect that the healing crystal will have on your body.

You can do this by focusing your intent on the crystal and thereby amplifying its own energy. A crystal that has been dedicated and programmed will be a lot more powerful and will be an effective tool in healing.

The method to program your crystal is very simple. In order to charge your crystal with the right intention, begin by holding the crystal in your hand and start sensing its energy. Because you have just cleansed your crystal, the energy you feel will be very strong. Keep your mind calm and have a positive attitude; quietly ask your energy to connect with that of the crystal. Even though your crystal does not have a life of its own, it has an energy that it emits through resonance. Once you feel that you have done enough sensing and feel connected to the crystal's energy, think of what you will be using your crystal for and then quietly ask the stone to act according to the way you want it to. You may feel the energy of the crystal increase. This indicates that your healing crystal has been programmed and is ready for use again.

Once your crystal has been charged with a specific intent, it will stay that way until it is cleansed and programmed again!

Final Words

Thank you for taking the time to read *'Crystal Healing: Revealed! The exciting secret to using powerful crystals to awaken your chakras, boost your energy and transform your life.'*

I hope this book has taught you about healing crystals are and the way they work. You have also learned how to choose and pick your own crystal and maintain it. And you know various techniques to heal your mind and body with the help of crystals.

Crystal healing is used as an alternative healing technique. This technique can be done by anyone if they are rightly guided and have the right mindset to perform it. It helps in the complete healing of mind, body and soul.

While these techniques help to improve your health and other aspects of your life, they don't create miracle strategies. Don't expect the change to happen overnight though; crystal healing takes effort and time.

Try not to focus on a lot of things simultaneously. Instead, try to heal one particular part of yourself at a time. Patience is a virtue that is very much needed with this type of healing.

I hope this book has helped you understand the basic concepts behind crystal healing and has guided you as to how to improve yourself holistically.

The next step is to apply what you have learned. To go out there, find the crystals you resonate with, and do your first crystal healing session. This can be a challenging process at times. We all have our moments of weakness. Take it one step at a time. And don't beat yourself up if you temporarily fall off track. Nobody is perfect! Success is simply a matter of getting up one more time than you fall.

I wish you success on your journey, and I hope you quickly experience the amazing benefits of crystal healing!

***

BONUS CHAPTER: What is Yoga

Below is the first chapter, called: 'What Is Yoga', from one of my other books, *'Yoga Bible For Beginners: 30 Essential Illustrated Poses For Better Health, Stress Relief and Weight Loss'*.

You have just learned how crystals can be used to heal body and mind. Did you know that there is a lot of synergy between crystal healing and practicing?

As you will see in the chapter below, yoga developed as a practice to help find – and maintain – balance, and live a healthy life. Practicing yoga regularly will not only increase your sense of wellbeing, but also amplify the effects of a crystal healing therapy session, and vice versa.

Enjoy!

***

"Yoga does not remove us from the reality or responsibilities of everyday life but rather places our feet firmly and resolutely in the practical ground of experience. We don't transcend our lives; we return to the life we left behind in the hopes of something better."

Donna Farhi

***Key Takeaway**: Yoga has been practiced for thousands of years. The word yoga means 'union'. It was originally designed as a path to reach enlightenment. As such, its primary focus was on transcending mind and body. In modern yoga, especially in the Western world, the word yoga has taken on a more literal meaning: a union between body and mind. Awareness is the most important aspect of yoga.*

Yoga is a practice that originated in India, with roots going back thousands of years. The word yoga means 'union'. Yoga was originally designed as a path to realize the true nature of one's self; or in other terms, enlightenment.

In the yoga tradition, yoga was understood to mean union between oneself and the origin of creation. In modern yoga, especially in the Western world, the word yoga has taken on a more literal meaning: a union between body and mind.

***

The History of Yoga

The practice of yoga originally focussed primarily on transcending the mind, not so much on the physical body, which is more common in modern yoga. In classical texts like Patanjali's Yoga Sutras, the focus is mostly on meditation, and hardly on asanas, or yoga poses.

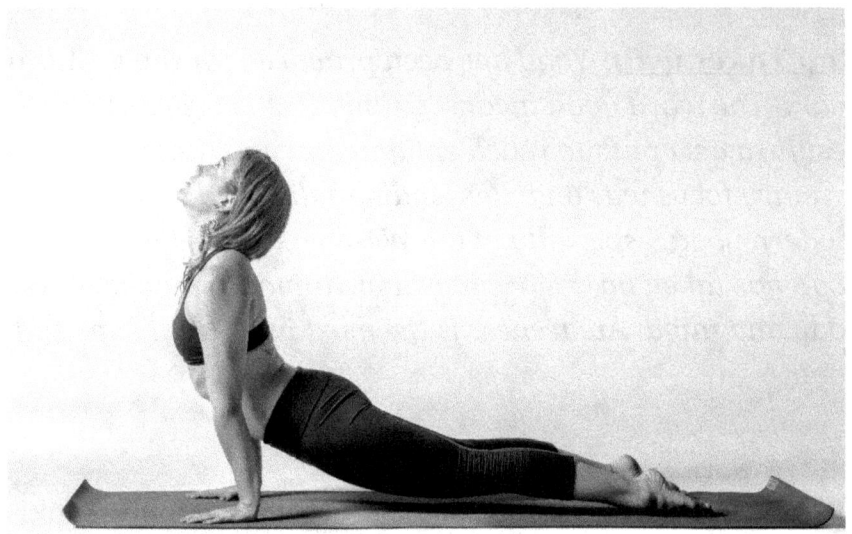

Over time, Tantra yoga developed, which accepted that this world is a manifestation of the ultimate reality. We have to accept our condition here, but we have to understand it differently, in a transfigured way. This practically means seeing the divine source in everything around you. Think of how a young girl explores the world around her. She can be completely captivated by the small wonders of this world, like the beautiful colors of a flower, or a beetle racing through the grass. We can all practice this in our daily lives.

Tantra yoga introduced a new relationship to the physical body. Where the ascetic paths saw the body and its desires as something that needed to be transcended, tantra yoga teaches that there is only one supreme reality, and it includes our bodies and our world. Consciousness and matter are not separate, but two ends of one undivided spectrum, like two poles of a single magnet. Hence, the body was seen as a temple of the divine which needed to be kept fit to prepare it for spiritual realization.

This led to the creation of Hatha yoga, which is a vast collection of exercises including asanas (poses), pranayama (control of prana, the subtle energetic streams in the breath), bandhas (body locks) and mudras (hand gestures). By practicing these exercises, in combination with meditation, the practitioner aimed to acquire self-knowledge and ultimately realize his or her true self.

However, it was not just a matter of doing the practice, and then expecting to automatically achieve self-realization. Ultimately, self-realization was a gift bestowed upon the practitioner by grace. Therefore, persistence in practice was no guarantee of enlightenment, and practice best went hand in hand with detachment to the outcome.

All physical yoga styles we see in Western yoga classes today use poses that originate from Hatha – and thus Tantra – yoga. Styles like Ashtanga, Vinyasa Flow, Power yoga or Yin yoga, to name only a few. A good analogy would be to compare Tantra yoga to water and the many different styles to drinks like coke, orange juice or coffee. Each drink has a different flavor, but its core ingredient is water.

Yoga was first introduced to the Western world when Swami Vivekananda set foot on American soil in 1893 to address the Parliament of Religions held in Chicago.

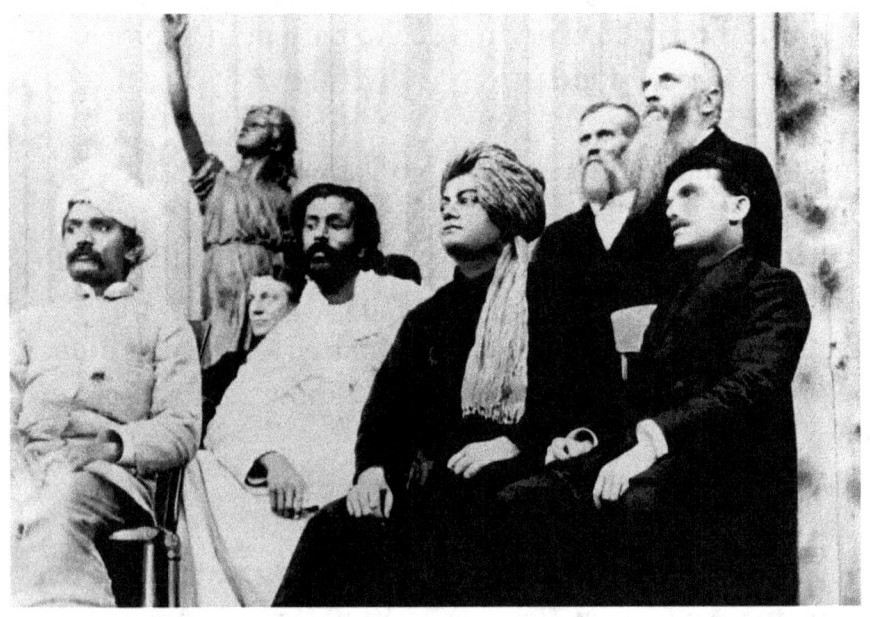

Swami Vivekananda at the Parliament of Religions held in Chicago

He brought a message of tolerance, which is as necessary today's world as it was in 1893. He shared the story of a frog who lived in a well. It had never left the well, and thought his well was the biggest water land of the world. Then, one day another frog came to visit his well. This frog came from the sea. When that frog of the sea told the frog of the well that the sea is much bigger than the well, he did not believe it and got angry, driving the frog of the sea away from his well. Vivekananda pointed out that people from different religions all sit in their own little well and think the whole world is their well.

***

Modern Yoga

In the early twentieth century, Yogananda moved to the US and brought his yoga teachings with him. In the 1940s, Indra Devi opened a yoga studio in Hollywood, after having studied with the famous India yoga guru Sri Tirumalai Krishnamacharya. He is considered the godfather of modern yoga. Krishnamachary was also the teacher of B.K. S. Iyengar, the founder of Iyengar yoga, and K. Pattabhi Jois, the founder of the popular Ashtanga yoga. These styles have become widely popular in the west, and have also inspired many other modern styles like Vinyasa, Bikram and Yin yoga.

Modern yoga revolves around uniting body and mind. This connection is often lost today, resulting in stress and obesity numbers rising through the roof. The body and mind are constantly interacting with each other. If you practice yoga, this will no longer be a mere intellectual concept, but something you will experience within. As the famous yoga teacher Swami Sivananda of Rishikesh said: *"An ounce of practice is worth more than a ton of theory."*

Many people are often very much 'in their head', so to speak, and less in touch with their body. Some even see their body simply as a mere means of getting their head into meetings! By focussing your attention on the breath or a body part, you restore the connection between mind and body. When you calm the body down with awareness, you also calm the mind.

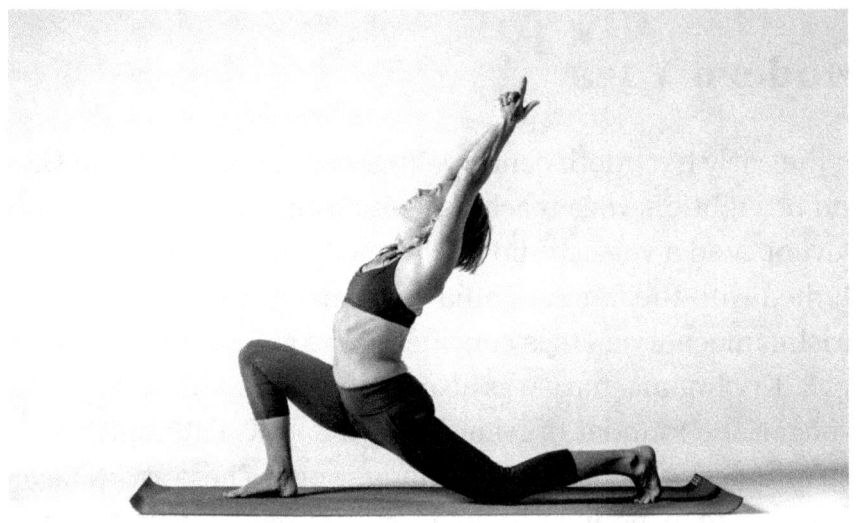

If there is one thing you remember from reading this book, let it be this:

<u>Awareness</u> *is the most important feature of yoga.*

When practicing the Standing Forward Bend, for example, it is completely irrelevant whether you can touch your toes or are only able to extend to the level of your knees. What matters is your state of mind. Flexibility will come.

Remember, unlike other forms of exercise, yoga is not about pushing far beyond your physical limitations, but about transforming the mind. If you compare yourself to those around you that are more flexible, this will negate the purpose of the exercise. When you feel challenged, or even tempted to give up, remember the purpose of yoga: to bring union between body and mind. Your mind is agitated now, but if you persevere and stick to the practice, you will be able to stop the fluctuations of the mind, at least temporarily. And you will feel so much better in your own body!

***

This is the end of this bonus chapter.

Want to continue reading?

Then get your copy of "Yoga Bible for Beginners" at your favorite bookstore!

Did You Like This Book?

If you enjoyed this book, I would like to ask you for a favor. Would you be kind enough to share your thoughts and post a review of this book? Just a few sentences would already be really helpful.

Your voice is important for this book to reach as many people as possible.

The more reviews this book gets, the more people will be able to find it and enjoy the incredible healing benefits that crystals can have.

***

IF YOU DID NOT LIKE THIS BOOK, THEN PLEASE TELL ME!

You can email me at **info@charicekiernan.com**, to share with me what you did not like.

Perhaps I can change it.

A book does not have to be stagnant, in today's world. With feedback from readers like yourself, I can improve the book. So, you can impact the quality of this book, and I welcome your feedback. Help make this book better for everyone!

Thank you again for reading this book and good luck with applying everything you have learned!

I'm rooting for you...

About The Author

Charice Kiernan is a certified yoga instructor with more than 10 years under her belt. She came into contact with yoga and meditation at a young age. After dedicating many years of her life to studying the profound Eastern teachings, combined with a daily yoga and meditation practice, she found an inner peace that she had never experienced before.

We often only truly understand something when we have to teach it to somebody else. This is how she found her calling: to share these wonderful teachings with the world.

By reading her books, you too can now get access to the amazing benefits and profound growth that yoga, meditation and mindfulness can bring to your life! Not just physically, but also mentally and emotionally.

True happiness comes from the ability to help others. This is why Charice feels very fortunate that she gets to share her passion with all of her students and readers. So many people have already reported feeling more energetic, happier and healthier! And this number is only growing.

So join Charice Kiernan on this journey of self-discovery, and become who you were destined to be.

To find out more, please visit **charicekiernan.com**.

By The Same Author

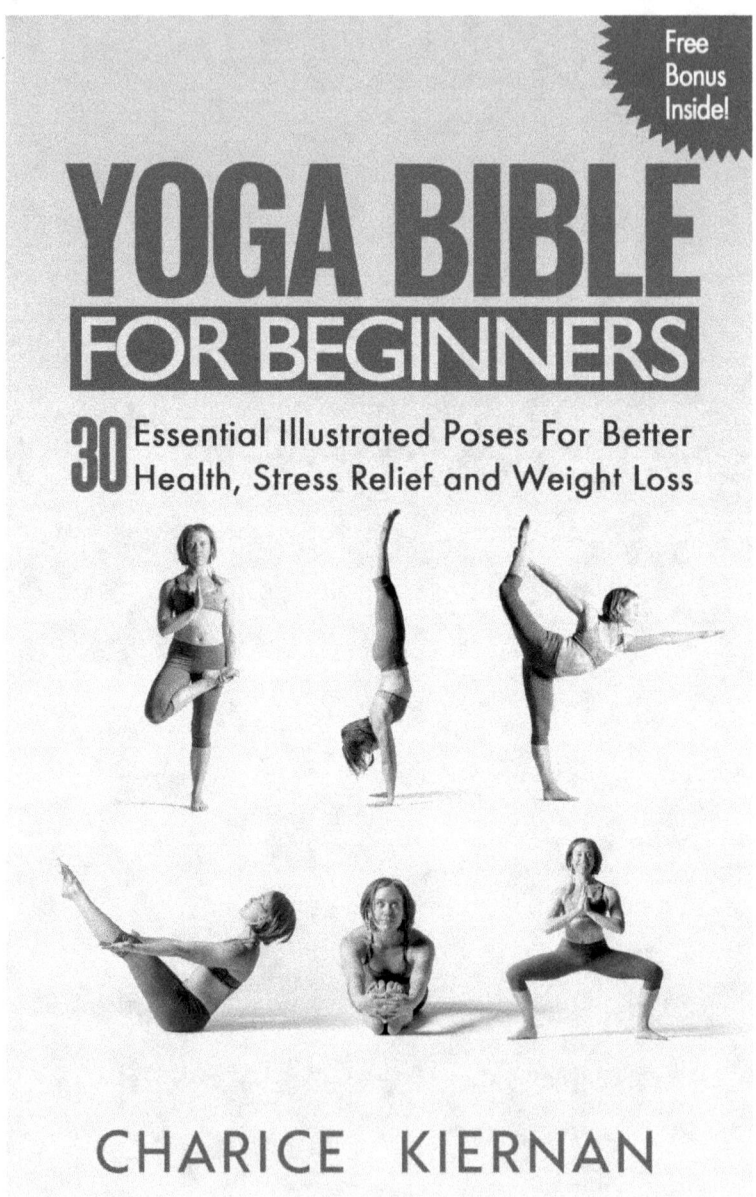

Notes